Paleo in a Snap

Mouth Watering Recipes for Busy Folks

Contents

About the Book

This book is written by following the Paleolithic diet guidelines. Learn about the Paleo diet in the introduction. Following the introduction, you will find a collection of tasty recipes that you can create in a short amount of time. From mouthwatering bacon wrapped scallops for an appetizer to delicious cookie dough popsicles for dessert, this book has great recipes with good nutrition. There are five sections of recipes including appetizers, breakfast, lunch, dinner and dessert. We hope you enjoy trying new combinations!

Introduction

The Paleolithic diet, also known as the caveman diet, is a nutritional plan based on foods from wild plants and animals. The diet is a modern adaptation to the pre-agriculture hunter-gatherers. All humans consumed this diet in the Paleolithic era that began 2.5 million years ago and continued until 10,000 years ago when the development of agriculture introduced grain-based diets. The theory of Paleolithic eating is that humans are still genetically adapted to the diet. It consists of meats, seafood, fresh fruits and vegetables.

Followers of this diet plan should consume 60% animal foods and 40% plant foods. The diet excludes cereal grains, legumes, dairy, refined sugar, processed foods, salt and refined vegetable oils. The framework includes higher intake of protein, fiber, potassium, omega 6 and 3 polyunsaturated/ monounsaturated fats, alkaline foods, vitamins, minerals, antioxidants and plant phytochemicals. By eliminating foods, the diet lowers carbohydrate intake, glycemic index, and sodium. Consuming this diet has shown to reduce health problems such as weight gain, cardiovascular disease, diabetes, metabolic syndrome, and gastrointestinal tract diseases, to name a few. Going back to these basics, has shown promise to optimize health, reduce disease and maintain a healthy weight.

Appetizers
Deviled Eggs

12 servings of 2 each
12 large eggs (boiled)
½ c. mayonnaise (Paleo)
1 tsp. mustard
Salt to taste
Pepper to taste
Cayenne pepper to taste
Curry powder to taste

Once your eggs are boiled, peel the shells and slice in half lengthwise. Then scoop the yolk out of each egg and put in a bowl. Mix together with the mustard and mayonnaise until smooth. Stir in seasonings to your taste liking. Spoon back into each egg half, cover and refrigerate for 2 hours. Serve.

Sweet Potato Crisps

6 Servings
3 large sweet potatoes (peel and slice)
¼ c. oil
Salt to taste
Cayenne pepper to taste

Preheat oven to 400 and line a baking sheet with parchment paper. In a medium bowl combine your oil, salt and cayenne pepper. Mix well. Coat each potato slice in the oil. Spread the potato slices out across the baking sheet and bake 15 minutes, flip and bake another 15 minutes.

Plantain Chips

4 Servings
2 unripe plantains
2 tbsp. olive oil
1 tsp. chili powder
½ tsp. ground cumin
1/8 tsp. cayenne pepper
½ tsp. sea salt

Heat up the oven to 400 and grease a cookie sheet. Slice the plantains into thin slices. In a medium bowl mix the oil and spices. Toss the plantains in the oil and seasoning mixture until well coated. Spread out on baking sheet and bake for 8 minutes, flip and bake for 8 minutes. Serve.

Yucca Fries

2 servings
1 large Yucca root
½ tsp. salt
1 tbsp. olive oil

Remove the skin of the yucca and slice into ½ inch length and width fries. Heat up the oven to 450 and bring a pot of water to a boil. Add the yucca to the boiling water and cook 30 minutes. Then remove the yucca and let it dry. Combine the oil and seasonings in a small bowl. Spread the yucca out on the baking sheet and pour the oil mixture to cover them. Bake 10 minutes, flip then bake 10 more minutes and serve.

Zucchini Bites

1 large zucchini (slice into rounds)
Olive oil
Salt to taste
Pepper to taste
Heat the oven to 225 and line with parchment paper. Spread out the zucchini, drizzle with olive oil and season. Bake 45 minutes, rotate and bake 45 more minutes. Check on them to get your desired crispiness.

Meatballs

1 lb. ground beef
1 medium carrot (finely grate)
1 yellow onion (chop)
1 large egg
Salt to taste
Pepper to taste

In a medium bowl, beat the egg until frothy and mix with the beef, carrot and onion. Add salt and pepper and combine well. Heat a large skillet over medium high heat with oil to fry. Then roll the meat into balls and add to the skillet.

Pumpkin Dip

12 Servings
6 c. organic pureed pumpkin
2 tbsp. caraway seeds
2 limes (for juice)
1 large lemon (for juice)
¼ c. olive oil (extra virgin)
1 tbsp. garlic (mince)
½ c. parsley (chopped)
1 tbsp. red chili pepper
Salt to taste
Pepper to taste

In a large skillet toast the seeds for about 10 minutes. Add the pumpkin and heat thoroughly. Then squeeze in the juice from the lime and lemons into a food processor and combine the garlic and pepper. Pulse until smooth. Stir in the garlic and chili pepper mixture and simmer for about 5 minutes so flavors can combine. Transfer to a large bowl and mix in the salt, pepper, parsley and olive oil. Mix well.

Pineapple Wrapped Bacon Bites

8 servings
1 lb. bacon strips (cut in half)
1 small pineapple (cut into bite size chunks)

Heat the oven to 375 and grease a baking sheet. Wrap each piece of pineapple in a half piece of a bacon strip and secure. Line them up on the baking sheet and bake 25 minutes.

Scallops Wrapped in Bacon

20 servings
10 strips of bacon (cut in half)
10 sea scallops (cut in half)
20 spinach leaves
1 lemon (cut in 4)

Heat the oven up to broiling and prepare a baking sheet. Place a spinach leave around each scallop and wrap a piece of bacon around that. Secure with a toothpick and line them up on the baking sheet. Broil 12 minutes, flipping half way through.

Breakfasts
Blueberry Pancakes with Bacon

2 servings
2 strips bacon (fry and drain)
2 large eggs
3 tbsp. water
1/8 c. coconut flour
Handful of blueberries

Break the bacon into bite size pieces. In a medium bowl, beat the eggs and mix them with flour, water and blueberries. Heat a large skillet over medium heat and drop the bacon in and then pour half the batter on top into a circle shape. Allow it to stiffen then flip it over and brown the other side. When finished remove it from the pan and cook the other half of the bacon and pancake.

Pumpkin Smoothie

1 serving
1 small under ripe banana
6 cubes of ice
½ c. pureed pumpkin
½ c. coffee (cold)
½ tsp. pumpkin pie seasoning
¼ tsp. vanilla extract
Cinnamon to taste

Add the banana, pumpkin, and coffee into a blender and pulse. Then add in the cubes of ice, seasoning, vanilla and cinnamon. Blend thoroughly and serve.

Banana Apple Porridge

2 servings
1/3 c. unsweetened almond milk
1.5 tbsp. finely ground flax seed
1 small ripe banana
1 chopped apple
½ c. pecans (processed)
½ c. blueberries (fresh)
½ tbsp. cinnamon
½ tsp. nutmeg

Mash the banana. Remove the skin from the apple and chop it. Heat a small sauce pan over low heat and combine the milk, banana and apple. Heat for about 2 minutes then add in the spices and flax seed. Stir over low heat for 8 minutes then add the nuts and berries. Pour between 2 bowls and enjoy.

Vegetable Egg Cups

6 servings
5 large eggs
2/3 c. grated zucchini
2/3 c. broccoli chopped
1 chopped green onion
2 tbsp. basil
1 tbsp. dried oregano
½ tsp. mustard (ground)
¼ tsp. baking powder
Ground pepper to taste

Heat up the oven to 350 and apply olive oil to each of the muffin cups. In a medium mixing bowl, beat the eggs until frothy and add the mustard, oregano, powder, pepper and salt. Then mix in the vegetables and basil. Combine well then pour into the muffin tin and bake 25 minutes.

Cereal

8 servings
1 c. sifted almond flour
2 tbsp. protein powder (vanilla)
¼ c. chia seeds
1 tsp. cinnamon
¼ c. coconut oil
¼ c. 100% pure cocoa
Honey to taste

Preheat the oven to 350 and line with parchment paper. In a medium bowl, mix together the flour, protein powder, seeds, cinnamon and cocoa. Combine well. Stir the oil in a separate bowl to get a smooth consistency then mix the dry mix with the oil. Add onto the baking sheet and bake 15 minutes. Top with honey, let cool and serve or store in an air tight container in the refrigerator.

Berry Muffins

12 servings
½ c. sifted coconut flour
½ tsp. sea salt
½ tsp. baking soda
½ tsp. baking powder
5 large eggs
2 eggs (yolks removed)
½ c. applesauce (no sweetener)
1 tsp. pure vanilla extract
½ c. almond butter
1 c. blueberries

In a large bowl mix together the flour, salt, baking soda and baking powder until well combined. In a separate bowl beat the eggs, egg whites, applesauce, vanilla and butter until smooth. Then mix into the flour mixture. It is best to use an electric mixer on high for about 5 minutes. Fold in the blueberries and disperse evenly. Divide the batter between the cups and bake 25 minutes.

Frittata

8 servings
1 lb. sausage
1 large yam (peeled and chopped into small cubes)
¾ onion (yellow diced)
¾ bell pepper (red, diced)
7 large eggs
Sea salt to taste
Pepper to taste

Heat up the oven to 400 and line a baking sheet with parchment paper then cover it with coconut oil. Bake the potatoes for 25 minutes. Heat a large skillet over medium high and add the onion, pepper and sausage. Crumble the sausage into small pieces and cook the whole combination for about 10 minutes. Once lightly browned and cooked through mix with the potatoes in a bowl. Break the eggs into a medium bowl and whisk until frothy. Then pour into the potato and skillet mixture. Grease the skillet with coconut oil and pour the frittata mixture in it. Cook 6 minutes then place in the oven and bake until browned and cooked through.

Pumpkin Raisin Muffin

2 Servings
1 small ripe banana
½ tbsp. melted coconut oil
½ tbsp. maple syrup
1 large egg
2 tbsp. coconut flour
1 tsp. baking powder
Salt to taste
½ tsp. ground cinnamon
2 tbsp. pumpkin puree
2 tbsp. crushed walnuts
2 tbsp. brown raisins

In a small sauce pan mash up the banana and heat over low. Mix in the oil and syrup and combine well. In a coffee mug combine the flour, powder, salt and cinnamon. Mix well and pour in the banana combination. Stir in the egg and pureed pumpkin. When smooth add raisins and nuts, disperse throughout and divide between two mugs. Microwave 2 minutes each. Sprinkle with cinnamon.

Granola

20 Servings
2 c. almonds
2 c. hazelnuts
1 c. cashews
1 c. Brazilian nuts
½ c. sunflower seeds
½ c. pumpkin seeds
1 c. unsweetened coconut flakes
2 tbsp. coconut flour
3 tbsp. chia seeds
¼ c. raisins
4 tbsp. melted coconut oil
3 ½ tbsp. pure maple syrup
1 tbsp. cinnamon
1 tbsp. pure vanilla extract
Salt to taste

Process all the nuts in a food processor then place in a large bowl. Mix them with the seeds then oil, vanilla and syrup and cover completely. Heat up the oven to 320 degrees and line a baking sheet with parchment paper. Pour the mixture on the baking sheet and bake 10 minutes before adding in the raisins to bake 10 minutes more. Cool in the fridge for 30 minutes then break up and serve or save in an air tight container.

Blueberry Cream Breakfast

4 pears (diced)
1 c. fresh blueberries
2 tbsp. melted coconut oil
1 tsp. ground cinnamon
1 can of coconut milk (full fat)
1 tsp. pure vanilla extract

Heat up the oven to 375 degrees and prepare a square 8 inch baking dish. Peel the pears and dice into ½ inch pieces. Combine the pears and blueberries in a bowl with cinnamon and coconut oil. Then pour into the baking dish and place foil over. Bake 20 minutes, remove the cover and bake 10 minutes. Top with the cream from the top of the coconut milk can along with vanilla.

Sweet and Spicy Bacon Strips

½ lb. bacon
½ c. pure maple syrup
½ tbsp. Dijon mustard
¼ tsp. cayenne pepper

Heat up the oven to 400 degrees and cover a baking sheet with foil. Combine syrup, mustard and pepper and dip the bacon slices in it. Then line on the baking sheet and bake 25 minutes.

Lunch
Taco Salad

Serves 2
1 lb. beef (ground)
1 red onion (diced)
Tomatoes (cherry)
Handful of spinach
1 head of romaine lettuce
1 plantain (yellow and black) sliced ¼ inch
1 tbsp. coconut oil
1 avocado (mashed)
Lime (for juice)

Melt the oil in a large skillet over medium high. Add the beef and brown thoroughly. Remove the beef, drain and set aside. Clean the skillet and add more coconut oil. Melt the oil over medium high heat, add the plantains and cook them until browned on both sides. Set aside. In a small bowl mash the avocado and mix with onion and juice. Cut up the lettuce and spread the spinach into two bowls. Add the beef on top of the lettuce. Split the guacamole between the two bowls. Add diced onions, halved tomatoes and plantain slices on top.

Brussel Sprouts and Apple Salad

Serves 3
12 Brussels sprouts
2 apples (peeled, cored and chopped)
1 small red onion (diced)
2 cloves of garlic (minced)
1 piece of ginger (1 inch)
2 tbsp. olive oil (extra virgin)
Salt to taste
Pepper to taste

Slice the ends of the sprouts off and chop up into strips. Combine it with the apples, onion, garlic and ginger. Mix well. Toss with juice, oil, salt and pepper.

Chicken Salad

Serves 4
4 grilled chicken breasts (sliced)
1 small onion (diced)
4 green onions (chopped)
3 celery stalks (chopped)
1 avocado
¼ c. water
1 tsp. olive oil
1 tsp. mustard
2 tsp. lemon juice
1 tsp. vinegar (apple cider)
¼ tsp. raw honey
Salt to taste
Pepper to taste

In a small bowl mash the avocado and combine with oil, mustard, water, lemon, vinegar, salt, pepper and honey. Stir and add to the food processor. Pulse until smooth. Dice up the chicken and stir the onions in with the avocado mixture. Serve.

Dinner
Beef Kabobs

Serves 4
2 lbs. beef
1 red bell pepper
1 yellow onion
Seasonings of choice

Heat up the oven to 450 and cover the baking sheet with coconut oil. Season the beef chunks, pepper and onions in the seasoning mixture. Chop the peppers and onions into squares. Thread them onto skewers with beef, onion, pepper and repeating.

Paleo Style Pizza

Serves 4
Crust:
1 lb. ground beef
1 clove of garlic minced
Red pepper crushed (to taste)
Chili powder to taste
Italian seasoning to taste
6 oz. tomato paste
Coconut oil
Toppings:
1 large sweet potato
1 head of broccoli
1 cauliflower
½ c. sun dried tomatoes
4 Brussels sprouts
4 oz. sliced mushrooms

Heat up the oven to 350 degrees .Start with the crust ingredients. Mix the seasonings into your ground beef. Prepare your 9 inch round baking dish by greasing it with coconut oil. Press the meat into the skillet and cover with the tomato sauce. Then chop up all the vegetables and put them on top. Bake for 60 minutes.

Chili Bowls

Serves 5
1 lb. beef hot dogs
1 tbsp. melted coconut oil
1 lb. beef (ground)
1 yellow onion (diced)
1 garlic cloves (crushed)
2/3 c. broth
1/3 c. tomato paste
2 tsp. pure cacao powder
2 tsp. chili
1 tsp. ground cumin
Salt to taste
Pepper to taste
Cinnamon to taste

In a large skillet over medium high heat, add the beef and allow it to brown. Add garlic and onion after about 5 minutes then continue to cook until the meat is cooked thoroughly. Once browned, add cacao, chili, cumin, salt, pepper and cinnamon. After the spices are mixed through the meat add the tomato and broth. Once it boils, reduce the heat to low. Simmer until it thickens for about 8 minutes then add sliced hot dogs. Cook 5 minutes and serve.

Pot Roast with Onions

Serves 5
3 lb. rib roast
2 c. red wine
¼ c. gluten free soy sauce
3 tbsp. olive oil
1 yellow onion chopped
6 chopped carrots
3 cloves of garlic minced
Pinch of dried basil
Pinch of dried oregano
Salt to taste
Pepper to taste

Marinate the rib roast in the soy sauce and wine overnight. Then heat a medium skillet with the olive oil over medium heat. Add the onions and allow them to caramelize. Then add the roast to a crock pot on high heat. Add all other ingredients and cook 7 hours.

Jambalaya

Serves 4
1 lb. shrimp (large, peeled)
2 chicken sausages
1 tbsp. olive oil (extra virgin)
15 oz. diced tomatoes
1 c. chicken broth
1 onion (diced)
1 tsp. paprika
1 tsp. cumin
Cayenne pepper to taste
Pepper to taste
Salt to taste
Splash of olive oil (extra virgin)
1 tsp. rice vinegar
1 head of cauliflower
3 cloves of garlic (minced)

Sauté the shrimp and sliced chicken sausages in a large skillet over medium high heat for 5 minutes. Next add in the onions, spices and tomatoes and sauté for 5 minutes. Next add the broth and cook until it boils, then reduce to low and cover. Process the cauliflower in a food processor until it is in small pieces. Heat olive oil and minced garlic in a medium sized pot and mix with the cauliflower, vinegar, salt and pepper. Scoop the cauliflower on to a plate and top with shrimp mixture.

Beef Curry

Serves 8
1 lb. beef stew meat
2 tbsp. melted coconut oil
1 bell pepper (red and sliced)
2 cloves of garlic (mince)
½ tsp. ginger (grate)
4 tbsp. curry paste
1 eggplant (cut into cubes)
1 c. peas (sugar snap)
2 cans coconut milk (full fat)

Heat up the coconut oil over medium and brown the outsides of the beef. Once thoroughly seared remove the beef from the pan and add the peppers and leeks. Season them with salt and pepper. Place the lid on until the vegetables soften up. Stir in the minced garlic, curry and ginger and simmer 5 minutes. Then add the peas, coconut milk and cubed eggplant. Cover, lower to low heat and simmer 5 minutes. Place the beef back in and cook over low for 30 minutes. Serve.

Cashew Chicken

Serves 3
2 c. cooked chicken breasts (cut into cubes)
¼ c. cashews
2 c. bell peppers (chopped)
2 c. processed cauliflower
1 small yellow onion diced
Chopped cilantro
2 tbsp. olive oil
Sauce:
2 tbsp. almond butter
1 tbsp. gluten free soy sauce
1 tbsp. olive oil
2 tbsp. water
1 clove of garlic (minced)
1 tsp. honey

Heat a skillet over medium heat and add the olive oil. Sauté the onion and peppers until they are browned. Then add the garlic and chicken. Sauté the processed cauliflower with olive oil over medium heat for 5 minutes. In a medium bowl mix together all sauce ingredients until well combined. Then add them in a large bowl with the chicken mixture and cauliflower. Serve and mix with nuts and cilantro.

Desserts
Cookie Dough Popsicles

9 Servings
1 c. unsweetened almond milk
1 tbsp. arrowroot powder
13.5 oz. coconut milk (full fat)
3 tbsp. palm sugar (raw coconut)
Salt to taste
2 tsp. pure vanilla extract
Dark chocolate chips

In a small bowl combine the arrowroot with the milk. Then add in the coconut milk, salt and coconut sugar, Heat in a medium saucepan over medium high heat. Once it hits a boil remove it from the heat. Once it has cooled all the way, pour in the vanilla. Fill Popsicle molds with the dark chocolate chips. Pour the milk mixture on top of the chocolate. Then pour a little bit more milk and sprinkle chocolate chips again. Insert the sticks and place in the freezer until solid.

Banana Chocolate Chip Brownies

5 servings
1 c. dark chocolate chips
¾ c. almond butter
2 large eggs
1 tsp. baking soda
Salt to taste
1 medium banana
1 c. almond flour
1/3 c. honey
1 tsp. pure vanilla extract

Heat up the oven to 350 and grease a baking dish. In a large bowl mix together all wet ingredients. Once smooth stir in the flour, baking soda and salt until smooth and no lumps. Bake 25 minutes then let cool down for about a half an hour. Then slice and serve.

Mini Apple Pies

12 servings
½ c. sifted coconut flour
½ tsp. sea salt
½ tsp. baking soda
1.2 tsp. baking powder
1 tsp. ground cinnamon
5 large eggs
2 eggs (eggs removed)
½ c. almond butter
1 tsp. pure vanilla extract
13 tbsp. raw honey
1 red apple (peeled, cored and chopped)
1 banana (mashed)

Heat up the oven to 350 and grease the muffin tins. In a medium bowl beat the eggs until frothy then add in all remaining ingredients excluding the apples. Once well combined and smooth, add in the apples. Then divide the mix between the muffin tins and bake 20 minutes. Cool and serve.

www.ingramcontent.com/pod-product-compliance
Lightning Source LLC
Chambersburg PA
CBHW080347290526

45791CB00009BA/2770